# Thyroid Disorders and Treatments: Underactive and Overactive Glands

## Understanding Hypothyroid and Hyperthyroid Conditions

By: James M. Lowrance © 2011

## *DEDICATION:*

To all of my fellow thyroid patients who take pride in being proactive in their treatments and in being self educated about their diseases.

*-Jim Lowrance*

**TABLE OF CONTENTS:**

## INTRODUCTION:

In this book (approximately 6,025 words in length), I have endeavored to inform the reader with all of the basics regarding hypothyroidism and hyperthyroidism, including causes, symptoms, diagnosis and treatments for each. I have dedicated slightly more information to hypothyroidism, due to it being present in approximately 80% of thyroid patients. Hyperthyroidism is addressed amply within the information that follows, as well.

Medical research estimates state that up to half of thyroid disease cases remain undiagnosed. It was my intention to provide facts, minus the fillers that can sometimes accompany information on these subjects. Many readers are simply looking for a good, general education on disorders of thyroid dysfunction and they are less-interested in detailed medical explanations or in numerous research study quotes. Certainly there are readers who enjoy those aspects and I have included this very type of information in other books I have authored.

5

In the chapters of this book that follow however, I will stick to the essential information that will help to educate readers with the important facts regarding hypothyroid and hyperthyroid conditions.

CHAPTER ONE:

## Understanding Hypothyroidism: Underactive Thyroid

(Hypothyroid Conditions)

## 1. Being Hypothyroid Means Thyroid Hormone Levels are Low

The "hypo" prefix, when applied to anything, means it has become deficient or lacking something that is essential to its adequacy or survival. In the case of "hypothyroidism" the term is referring to a gland that no longer manufactures and distributes sufficient/adequate levels of thyroid hormones. The gland is either damaged, diseased or being hindered by something that is secondary to it (something not directly within the gland).

The "thyroxine" hormone, is the "T4", manufactured by the thyroid gland and its abbreviated-name comes from the fact that it contains 4 iodine hormones.

In addition to playing a role in keeping bodily
metabolism at the proper level; meaning the rate
at which the body burns energy-producing fuels
(i.e. food, water and oxygen) it is also a precursor
to the T3 thyroid hormone, which contains 3
iodine molecules. With the aid of essential
proteins and enzymes, T4 which is in larger
reserve within the body than is T3 but being less
powerful, drops one of its iodine molecules, to
become the higher-strength hormone.

The T3 hormone, also called "triiodothyronine",
utilizes iodine by converting it into its own
metabolism-regulating properties, after absorbing
it from things in the diet. Many foods contain this
essential element but in the less industrialized
countries of the world, where iodized table sale is
not available or adequate nutritional foods, iodine
deficiency hypothyroidism is more common. T3
is reported by medical sources to be from 5 to 10
times more powerful than is the T4 hormone, in
spite of it containing one-less iodine molecule.

When either or both of these hormones become
low within the body, symptoms of a hypothyroid
state will begin to develop.

8

## 2. Hypothyroidism causes Slowed Bodily Metabolism

As mentioned, the metabolism provides ongoing energy for the body at the proper level. If thyroid hormones become low, energy-levels drop and underactive thyroid symptoms will begin to develop. This will affect all systems within the body including digestion, other hormone levels (i.e. the adrenal, sex and glucose-regulating ones) and cardiopulmonary functions. These will all become slowed-down and as a result, mental and emotional aspects of an affected individual, will also experience negative effects.

The symptoms of hypothyroidism can include the following:

* Constipation
* Dry Skin and brittle hair
* Loss of libido
* Slowed heart rate and breathing
* Inability to fully concentrate
* Depression

While the last symptom listed, is depressed mood, hypothyroid patients can experience anxiety symptoms in some cases as well. This may be due to other hormone levels within the body rising, as the body attempts to compensate for the low metabolism. Anxiety may also be experienced in those who develop autoimmune hypothyroidism (Hashimoto's disease) because a condition known as "Hashitoxicosis" can be a precursor to the onset of progressive hypothyroidism and which causes a temporary overactive thyroid gland (transient thyrotoxicosis).

## 3. How TSH Reacts to Hypothyroidism

TSH or "Thyroid Stimulating Hormone", is a hormone coming from a major endocrine gland found near the center of the brain called the "pituitary". It is released from this command-center and sent to the thyroid, to stimulate adequate/normal levels of thyroid hormones to be manufactured and distributed.

When thyroid hormones become low for any reason, the TSH is increased by the pituitary gland and if they become high for any reason, it will be decreased to compensate for this as well.

These scenarios, will allow levels of the hormone, that are blood-tested for, to show up as abnormally high or low, which can then help an observing doctor to know if hypothyroidism or hyperthyroidism (overactive) has developed or is beginning to develop. The hormone can usually detect either condition, very early and usually even before the thyroid hormone levels fall outside of normal values.

## 4. Underactive Thyroid from Autoimmunity

As previously mentioned, "Hashimoto's thyroiditis" is the term most often used to describe hypothyroidism that has developed due to "thyroid autoimmunity". This is a term used for the condition, in which the immune system attacks the thyroid gland, via auto-antibodies it creates, once recognizing it as an intruder in the body that needs to be eradicated/destroyed. Medical experts have yet to understand fully, as to why the immune system attacks a natural part of the body, when its job is rather to kill-off any viruses, allergens or bacteria but some possible triggers may include lifetime viruses in the body, environmental toxins and nutritional deficiencies.

The causes may vary between each person who develops the disease.

The two main thyroid antibodies that are found present in the bodies/blood of patients with Hashimoto's disease, include the "Anti-Thyroid Peroxidase" (TPO) and the "Anti-Thyroglobulin" (TG). These attack either or both of the proteins called "Thyroid Peroxidase" and "Thyroglobulin", which are essential to the production of thyroid hormones.

## 5. The Other Causes of Hypothyroid Conditions

In addition to thyroid autoimmunity, hypothyroid conditions can occur in people whose pituitary glands have stopped functioning properly (usually due to a tumor within the gland) and this results in a condition of low TSH-availability called "Central Hypothyroidism". Women can become hypothyroid during pregnancy (gestational) and babies can be born hypothyroid (congenital). People whose thyroid glands are partially missing or damaged by things such as traumatic accidents, surgical thyroidectomies or excessive radiation can develop hypothyroidism as well.

If an underactive thyroid, is due to a condition within the gland itself, this is referred to as "primary hypothyroidism", while "secondary" causes affect the gland indirectly (i.e. non-thyroid diseases, nutritional deficiencies and traumatic stress). More on the "causes" of underactive thyroid conditions will be addressed in CHAPTER FIVE, in which I provide a "quiz" on the subject.

## 6. Treating Hypothyroidism

The goal in treating hypothyroidism, is to replace the low levels of hormones, via a daily prescribed dosing of them and to monitor the treatment via regular-interval blood testing to re-evaluate the ongoing levels. This will both alleviate symptoms and restore normal bodily metabolism. A qualified treating doctor can determine the type of thyroid hormone replacement, that is best suited for each individual patient (i.e. T4 only and combination T4/T3 prescriptions), as well as the size doze that is ultimately needed for adequate or optimal treatment (dose-adjustments are usually needed during the first few months of therapy). More regarding treatments will be addressed in CHAPTER THREE.

CHAPTER TWO:

## Understanding Hyperthyroidism: Overactive Thyroid

(Hyperthyroid Conditions)

Conditions of hyperthyroidism, affect about 20% of people with thyroid disease. In this article, I will discuss the causes, symptoms and treatments for overactive thyroid glands.

The following 6 points help us to understand hyperthyroid conditions.

## 1. Hyperthyroidism means Thyroid Hormone Levels are High

With hyperthyroid conditions, the major thyroid hormones, being the T4 and T3, become elevated in the body. Since these hormones are what set the rate of metabolism, meaning the speed at which the body utilizes energy from things consumed (i.e. food, water and oxygen); this causes the metabolic rate to run abnormally high.

Either or both of these major thyroid hormones will elevate as the thyroid gland becomes overactive in producing them. Other medical terms for this condition are "thyrotoxicity" and "thyrotoxicosis".

## 2. Hyperthyroid Symptoms Due to Increased Metabolism

Once levels of the thyroid hormones, reach values that are above normal, the symptoms of increased metabolism will begin to occur, which can include nervousness and anxiety, rapid heart rate (tachycardia), diarrhea, high levels of energy followed by fatigue, weight loss, increased appetite, hair loss, oily skin, excessive sweating and inflammation in the eyes (Thyroid Eye Disease). As the condition worsens, a person may also begin to experience loss of muscle mass, osteoporosis (bone loss) and malabsorption of nutrients in the digestive tract (malnutrition). Chronic, untreated hyperthyroidism can also result in heart arrhythmias and disease of the heart muscle.

## 3. TSH Decreases with Hyperthyroidism

As the pituitary gland in the brain, which stimulates the thyroid gland, begins to recognize that it is overactive; it will send-out less TSH hormone (Thyroid Stimulating Hormone). This will cause levels of the hormone to drop, which can be found via blood lab testing. If a lab range for example, has a normal value of "0.3 to 4.0", the TSH in a hyperthyroid person will drop to the lower end of the range or it will be flagged below normal (noted as abnormally low on the lab result). In some cases the TSH will begin to lower, even before the T3 and/or T4 levels are flagged high, which also occurs as the condition progresses.

## 4. Hyperthyroidism can be Autoimmune in Nature

According to published medical statistics, approximately 85% of hyperthyroid cases, are caused by an autoimmune condition called Graves' disease. The National Institute of Health in the U.S. states that up to 3% of the American population has Graves' disease.

It affects females from 5 to 10 times more commonly than males. It is more common in people who are middle-aged but it can also occur in adolescents and in the elderly. The main antibody, sent from the immune system, to the thyroid gland that results in its over-activity in producing excessive hormones, is called "Thyroid Stimulating Immunoglobulin" (TSI). This antibody mimics the action of TSH, in stimulating this activity that results in Graves' disease and hyperthyroidism.

## 5. Other Causes of Hyperthyroidism

In addition to thyroid autoimmunity, other causes of hyperthyroid conditions, can include hot nodules, which are small tumors within the gland that excrete thyroid hormones (also referred to as "toxic adenoma"), excessive iodine in the diet (i.e. too much kelp or supplements/drugs containing high levels) and viral illnesses that settle in the thyroid gland, resulting in viral thyroiditis (temporary inflammation in the gland, resulting in short-term hyperthyroidism).

Hypothyroid patients, who are administered hormone replacement therapy for their under-active thyroid glands, can become hyperthyroid by taking doses that are too high. Some hypothyroid patients with autoimmune thyroiditis (Hashimoto's thyroiditis), experience transient, short-term hyperthyroidism as their disease is first developing, which is called "Hashitoxicosis".

People with Graves' disease, often have a "toxic goiter", meaning their thyroid gland is both enlarged and secreting excessive amounts of thyroid hormones. If a person has both a goiter and hot nodules causing hyperthyroidism, they may be termed as having a "toxic multi-nodular goiter" (Plummer's disease).

## 6. Hyperthyroid Treatments

If a person has Graves' disease causing their hyperthyroidism, this will usually result in the need to eventually remove the thyroid gland surgically (thyroidectomy) or in the need to destroy the gland via a procedure called "Radioactive Iodine Ablation" (RAI).

18

The RAI procedure is designed to burn the gland into nonexistence by controlled radiation that is mixed into an iodine dose and administered to the hyperthyroid patient under medical supervision.

It can take several weeks following an RAI procedure, for all thyroid tissue in the body to be fully eradicated. Once this occurs, the patient will become hypothyroid (lack of thyroid hormone in the body) and they will require a daily dose of hormone replacement therapy, as a lifelong treatment thereafter. In the case of hot nodules, only part of the gland containing the tumor may need to be surgically removed, which is referred to as a "partial or subtotal thyroidectomy".

Some doctors will attempt to control hyperthyroidism caused by Graves' disease, through administration of "anti-thyroid drugs", which can block the excessive production of thyroid hormones. Patients may also need to be placed on doses of beta-blocker medications that help to control hypertension and tachycardia, if needed. If these treatments do not successfully control symptoms, thyroid removal options would then be considered.

*Thyroid Disorders and Treatments: Underactive and Overactive Glands*

Temporary types of hyperthyroidism, caused by viral thyroiditis, usually require no treatment, other than bed-rest, medication for fever and simply allowing the virus to run its course, so that thyroid function can return to normal.

Hyperthyroidism and its causes are diagnosed through blood testing of the TSH and thyroid hormones and with thyroid imaging tests.

## CHAPTER THREE:

## Understanding Thyroid Hormone Replacement Therapies

(The Treatment of Hypothyroid Conditions)

Hypothyroidism affects an estimated 10% of Americans but some medical research groups believe that this number is likely twice as high, due to half of those affected, remaining undiagnosed.

When hypothyroid conditions develop, treatment must be administered to prevent a chronic worsening of the condition, which can eventually lead to myxedema coma and/or death.

Moderate to severe hypothyroidism can also cause other problems in the body, if left untreated, including increasing weight gain, fluid retention (edema), worsening depression, high cholesterol and heart disease.

## Thyroid Supplements versus Hormone Replacement

While some manufacturers of thyroid boosting supplements, would have you to believe that these natural remedies will reverse or treat hypothyroidism, this is not true if they contain no thyroid hormone. The Federal Drug Administration (FDA) will not permit the adding of actual thyroid hormones to non-prescription supplements and so thyroid booster supplements cannot treat cases of true hypothyroidism, which occurs in diseased thyroid glands. In non-diseased glands, it is possible that some of these supplements do boost thyroid function to some degree but when overt (full blown) deficiency in thyroid hormones is present, there is no substitute for replacing them via prescribed hormone therapy, administered by a qualified medical doctor.

## Types of Thyroid Hormone Replacement Drugs

Most hypothyroid patients are prescribed T4 medications to restore bodily metabolism that begins to run low as a result of the condition.

This hormone, also called "levothyroxine" is usually prescribed in the synthetic form, such as the name-brand called Synthroid™. The hormone will then also convert into another major thyroid hormone called the T3 (triiodothyronine), via the available globulins, enzymes and proteins that are present in the body. Much of this conversion process occurs within the liver and kidneys.

Some hypothyroid patients are believed to have a problem with converting T4 into the also essential T3 due to a lack of these conversion elements in the body (impaired conversion). This may be discovered when the hormone replacement is monitored via blood lab tests, of these two hormones.

When this failure to convert is found to be occurring, a treating-doctor may switch patients to a T3 and T4 combination medication, such as the brand Armour™ (natural) or the brand Thyrolar™ (synthetic) or they may simply add a T3 medication to the therapy, such as the synthetic brand Cytomel™.

## How Hypothyroid Treatment is Monitored

As a hypothyroid patient takes their prescribed, daily dose of replacement hormones, this will cause levels in the body to increase, until they reach normalized states (euthyroid). This can however take several dose adjustments to be made, over a period of several months, before optimized levels are achieved. The method for monitoring the treatment is by repeat blood testing, ordered at regular intervals of 6 to 8 weeks between dose changes. Once the proper level is reached, a doctor may only require patients to be retested, two or three times yearly.

The tests that are ordered usually include the TSH, the T4 and the T3. The TSH (Thyroid Stimulating Hormone) is actually a pituitary hormone that stimulates thyroid function and that decreases when thyroid hormones (T4 and T3) increase in the body and increases when they become lower in the body. For example, an abnormally high TSH indicates hypothyroidism or under-treated hypothyroid cases and an abnormally low TSH indicates hyperthyroidism or over-treated hypothyroid cases.

The opposite is true of the T4 and T3, which both decrease with hypothyroidism and they increase with hyperthyroidism.

## How Patients can help with their Treatment

Hypothyroid patients should take their daily hormone dose, as directed by their doctors and they should not make adjustments to the amount taken, unless approved, following a check up or blood lab testing.

The dose should be taken first thing upon waking, mornings and on an empty stomach to allow-for optimal absorption through the digestive tract and it should also be taken with a full glass of water. Breakfast should be delayed if-possible for at least 30 minutes and preferably for an hour after dosing.

Foods containing high-fiber content, should be avoided for at least two hours following the morning dose and any supplements containing calcium or iron, should be taken about 6 hours afterward, to also prevent malabsorption of the hormones.

25

A hypothyroid patient should not switch from a name-brand thyroid hormone, to a generic version, without the knowledge of their doctor. Even if the same amount of T4 and/or T3 is listed on a prescription generic, to be contained in each pill, as is contained in a major brand, there can still be differences in the potency. This can be due to differences in the fillers used in each drug and in whether it is animal-derived (dessicated) or synthetic (lab produced).

Thyroid hormone replacement therapy can resolve the symptoms of hypothyroidism and restore a better quality of life to patients.

## CHAPTER FOUR:

**Is Fibromyalgia Common in Treated
Autoimmune Hypothyroidism?**
(Chronic Muscle Pain in Hypothyroid Patients)

Many patients with both hypothyroidism and
hyperthyroidism, commonly complain to their
doctors about chronic muscle pain. This is a
definition of "Fibromyalgia", being co-morbid to
thyroid disease (associated with it and possibly
stemming from it). It is however, a more common
finding in hypothyroid patients, even after they
have undergone thyroid hormone correction
therapies.

Why would Fibromyalgia Syndrome (FMS) be
found to be so common among patients diagnosed
with thyroid diseases? According to medical
research that has been conducted in this area,
which has studied thyroid patients, FMS may be a
direct result of "thyroid auto-antibodies". These
are the cells produced and sent from the immune
system, to eradicate natural proteins and enzymes
within the thyroid gland. It is yet to be understood
by medical researchers, as to why this occurs.

It is evident to them however, that the immune system is recognizing these natural substances that play a factor in the production of thyroid hormones, as enemies to the body. This misguided identification of essential thyroid substances, causes damage to the hormone production system, so that hormone-imbalances occur, resulting in either hypothyroidism (an under-active thyroid) or hyperthyroidism (an overactive thyroid).

In hypothyroidism, the two main thyroid proteins that are attacked by auto-antibodies, are the "thyroidperoxidase" and the "thyroglobulin". Because of this misguided attack against these proteins, the auto-antibodies are referred to as the "anti-thyroidperoxidase" (abbreviated - "TPO") and the "anti-thyroglobulin" (abbreviated "TG"). In the case of hyperthyroid patients (those with "Graves' Disease"), an additional auto-antibody will manifest, called "Thyroid Stimulating Immunoglobulin". This later-mentioned immune cell (Abbreviated "TSI"), mimics the action of a pituitary gland hormone called "Thyroid Stimulating Hormone" (TSH). This is what results in the over-production of thyroid hormones or "hyperthyroidism".

28

Hypothyroid patients on the other hand, will see the TPO and TG auto-antibodies become the predominant ones in their autoimmune thyroid disease, which is referred to as "Hashimoto's thyroiditis". In this case, the immune system attack, renders the thyroid gland unable to produce adequate amounts of thyroid hormones to keep bodily-metabolism (cellular energy) at an adequate level. It rather remains at a lower-than-normal level, which is referred to as "hypothyroidism.

Both hyperthyroidism and hypothyroidism have treatments available, to adequately restore bodily-metabolism to normal levels. Treatments can actually accomplish this to optimal levels in some cases (e.g. hyperthyroid patients often have thyroidectomies - surgical thyroid gland removal). The auto-antibodies that remain present and that are not eradicated with treatment for hypothyroid patients (treatment consists of thyroid hormone supplementation, rather that thyroidectomy), may result in FMS symptoms. It is not fully understood as to why this is the case but it is understood that auto-antibodies of any kind, have the potential to cause varied degrees of chronic inflammation within the body.

This inflammation from thyroiditis, may prove to be the factor involved in causing FMS symptoms in hypothyroid patients. Medical researchers continue to study this aspect. Hopefully, they will find definitive reasons for the strong association of FMS to autoimmune hypothyroidism, that can remain after treatment of thyroid hormone deficiencies.

CHAPTER FIVE:

**Types of Hypothyroidism Quiz - - -**
(Test Your Knowledge about Hypothyroid
Types/Causes)

For those of you who enjoy quizzes, I have put
this one together for you. But, to increase your
chances of achieving a higher score, I am
providing this article that somewhat reviews and
adds more detail to information that was
discussed in CHAPTER ONE and that will be on
the quiz-subject (a brief run-down of hypothyroid
types).

The questions the quiz is comprised-of will be
posted at the end of this article and the correct
answers to them will be revealed afterward as
well (each correct answer is worth 10 points). The
quiz title is "Types of Hypothyroidism" and
following below are brief descriptions of those
that will be covered, although not necessarily in
the same order that will be reflected in the quiz-
questions.

## A Brief Run Down of Hypothyroid Types (To Prepare for Your Quiz) ---

As has been discussed in previous chapters, hypothyroidism is the term for a low functioning thyroid gland. While the different terms briefly-discussed below, have specific meanings and uses, there are times that they may crossover -- meaning two or more terms may sometimes apply to a particular case or type of hypothyroidism.

When women experience low thyroid hormone after pregnancy and following giving birth, the term for this type of underactive thyroid, is "postpartum hypothyroidism". This type happens in about 10% of new mothers and for some, it improves without treatment. Others may require short-term treatment with thyroid hormone replacement therapy. If the hypothyroidism that is triggered is the autoimmune type, the treatment for it will likely be life-long. This permanent type of hypothyroidism caused by thyroid autoimmunity is called "Hashimoto's thyroiditis" and pregnant women have a slightly higher susceptibility to developing this permanent condition.

One common acquired type of hypothyroidism that occurs in countries where diets are low in iodine is referred to as "iodine deficiency hypothyroidism". This type is rare in industrialized countries, and so is more common in those considered to be "third world countries" (less developed and less industrialized – usually lacking iodized salt).

When the cause of hypothyroidism, originates from within the gland itself, the term for this type is "primary hypothyroidism". The most common cause originating within the thyroid gland is disease processes, such as Hashimoto's thyroiditis. It would however, still be considered primary hypothyroidism even if it is due to a damaged gland. For example, a person whose gland is injured in an accident or damaged due to excessive exposure to radioactivity can become hypothyroid. The term "secondary hypothyroidism" on the other hand, means the gland is under-functioning due to another cause. This can be anything that affects the thyroid gland from outside of it, rather than it being a problem from within the gland itself.

There is also a type of hypothyroidism that is caused by a failure of the brain-center glands that regulate the thyroid (levels of hormone production). The two major glands in the brain that help regulate thyroid function are the hypothalamus and pituitary glands. The hypothalamus stimulates the pituitary, to produce TSH (thyroid stimulating hormone) and in response, the pituitary sends TSH to the thyroid gland to stimulate it. If a failure occurs within communication between these glands, it can cause the thyroid to under-function, which is referred to as "Central hypothyroidism".

Lastly, the more powerful T-3 thyroid hormone can become low in the body due to a lack of its production by the thyroid gland. This can be due to a temporary imbalance of "T-4 to T-3 conversion" (too much inactive "Reverse T-3" is being made from T-4, rather than "active T-3"). This type of hypothyroidism, is referred to by several different synonymous names. These include: Wilson's Temperature Syndrome, Sick Euthyroid Syndrome and Low T-3 Syndrome. It is often temporary and can be corrected by short term T-3 hormone replacement therapy.

\* \* \* \* \* \* \* \* \* \* \* \* \* \* \* \* \* \* \* \* \* \* \* \* \* \*

*Are you ready to take the "Types of Hypothyroidism" quiz?*

*Try it!...Give yourself a score of 10 points for each <u>correct</u> <u>answer</u> (revealed at the end):*

Question 1 of 10:

**What does "Primary Hypothyroidism" mean?**

(A.) The hypothyroidism originates from the brain.
(B.) The Hypothyroidism originates from an illness.
(C.) The hypothyroidism originates from the feet.
(D.) The hypothyroidism originates from within the thyroid gland.

Question 2 of 10:

**What does "Secondary Hypothyroidism mean?**

(A.) The hypothyroidism is caused by a disease.
(B.) The hypothyroidism is caused by failure of another gland in the body.
(C.) The hypothyroidism is caused by a medication that is being taken.
(D.) All of the above.

Question 3 of 10:

**What is "Central Hypothyroidism"?**

(A.) It is caused by standing in Grand Central Station.
(B.) It is caused due to the thyroid gland not sitting dead-center in the throat.
(C.) It is caused by reaching the center of a tootsie roll pop.
(D.) It is caused by failure of the brain-center glands (pituitary and/or hypothalamus).

Question 4 of 10:

**Which disease listed below causes "Autoimmune Hypothyroidism"?**

(A.) Addison´s Disease.
(B.) Hashimoto´s thyroiditis.
(C.) Insulin Resistance.
(D.) Athlete´s Foot.

Question 5 of 10:

**Which type of hypothyroidism is most common?**

(A.) Central Hypothyroidism.
(B.) Secondary Hypothyroidism.
(C.) Primary Hypothyroidism.
(D.) Mr. Magoo´s Hypothyroidism.

Question 6 of 10:

**When the body is converting too much of the T-4 thyroid hormone into "Reverse T-3", rather than active T-3, resulting in low T-3 hypothyroidism, what is this type called?**

(A.) Wilson´s Temperature Syndrome.
(B.) Sick Euthyroid Syndrome.
(C.) Low T-3 Syndrome.
(D.) All of the above.

Question 7 of 10:

**If a person´s thyroid gland is damaged in an accident, resulting in hypothyroidism, which type would this be?**

(A.) Primary Hypothyroidism.
(B.) Autoimmune Hypothyroidism.
(C.) Low T-3 Syndrome.
(D.) Secondary Hypothyroidism.

Question 8 of 10:

**Hypothyroidism that develops due to pregnancy is referred to by which name?**

(A.) Wilson´s Temperature Syndrome.
(B.) Nature´s Revenge.
(C.) Postpartum Hypothyroidism.
(D.) Hashimoto´s.

Question 9 of 10:

**The word "Hypothyroidism" actually refers to which condition below?**

(A.) A low functioning thyroid gland.
(B.) An inconsiderate husband.
(C.) An enlarged thyroid gland.
(D.) A high function adrenal gland.

Question 10 of 10:

**The acquired type of primary hypothyroidism called "Iodine Deficiency Hypothyroidism" is caused by which of the problems listed below?**

(A.) A lack of chocolate in the diet.
(B.) Drinking too many soda pops.
(C.) Use of cell phones while driving.
(D) Lack of iodine in the diet.

\* \* \* \* \* \* \* \* \* \* \* \* \* \* \* \* \* \* \* \* \* \* \* \* \*

*The Correct Answers Are:*

(1.) **What does "Primary Hypothyroidism" mean?**

CORRECT ANSWER "D": It is referred to by this name because it originates from "within the thyroid gland".

**(2.) What does "Secondary Hypothyroidism mean?**

CORRECT ANSWER "D": "All of the above" – Secondary Hypothyroidism can be <u>any cause</u> that is not directly due to failure of the gland itself.

**(3.) What is "Central Hypothyroidism"?**

CORRECT ANSWER "D": It is called Central Hypothyroidism because the thyroid gland failure is due to a problem within "the brain-center" (master glands that regulate the thyroid).

**(4.) Which disease listed below causes "Autoimmune Hypothyroidism"?**

CORRECT ANSWER "B": "Hashimoto´s thyroiditis".

**(5.) Which type of hypothyroidism is most common?**

CORRECT ANSWER "C": "Primary Hypothyroidism" - The type caused by a problem within the thyroid gland itself is the most common.

**(6.) When the body is converting too much of the T-4 thyroid hormone into "Reverse T-3", rather than active T-3, resulting in low T-3 hypothyroidism, what is this type called?**

CORRECT ANSWER "D": "All of the above" - When the T-3 hormone becomes low due to over-production of Reverse T-3, it can be referred to by <u>any of the names listed</u>, depending upon the cause.

**(7.) If a person's thyroid gland is damaged in an accident, resulting in hypothyroidism, which type would this be?**

CORRECT ANSWER "A": Even if hypothyroidism results from injury to the gland, it is referred to as "Primary Hypothyroidism" because the problem originates within the damaged gland.

**(8.) Hypothyroidism that develops due to pregnancy is referred to by which name?**

CORRECT ANSWER "C": The answer is "Postpartum Hypothyroidism" meaning it follows within the mother, after giving birth.

**(9.) The word "Hypothyroidism" actually refers to which condition below?**

CORRECT ANSWER "A": Hypothyroidism is a term referring to "a low functioning thyroid gland".

**(10.) The acquired type of primary hypothyroidism called "Iodine Deficiency Hypothyroidism" is caused by which of the problems listed below?**

CORRECT ANSWER "D": The answer is "lack of iodine in the diet".

\* \* \* \* \* \* \* \* \* \* \* \* \* \* \* \* \* \* \* \* \* \* \* \* \*

So, how did you score on this quiz?

CHAPTER SIX:

## Understanding Thyroid Gland Biopsy and Imaging Tests

(When Blood Testing doesn't Tell the Whole Story)

While blood testing is the single most commonly used method to detect thyroid hormone imbalance, other medical lab tests can also be needed to identify thyroid disease processes.

The two ways in which a diseased thyroid gland can be more thoroughly analyzed are through studies if tissue samples from the gland (biopsy) and by taking detailed images of the gland (imaging tests).

## Fine Needle Aspiration (Tissue Biopsy)

When a thyroid gland has suspicious looking nodules within it (small tumors) that might contain malignancy, meaning cancer cells, with papillary and follicular thyroid cancers being the most common types, a biopsy sample might be extracted from the gland for analysis.

This can either be done surgically or by use of a less invasive procedure called a "fine needle aspiration" (FNA).

The FNA is performed usually as an in-office, out-patient procedure, using a hypodermic needle to extract tissue from a specific area of the thyroid gland. If for example, a nodule is of a significant size or has a firmness to it (solid nodule), a doctor with experience in FNA, can extract a sample of tissue from the tumor itself, to rule-out or confirm the presence of malignant cells.

The procedure can also detect the presence of thyroid autoimmunity, such as Hashimoto's thyroiditis -- a condition in which the thyroid gland is being destroyed by auto-antibodies from the immune system, also referred to as "chronic lymphocytic thyroiditis". This disease is at-times elusive to detection by blood testing analysis, especially during early stages of the disease and the FNA can detect it, despite negative auto-antibodies in a patient's blood.

## Thyroid Imaging Tests

When doctors examine patient's thyroid glands by palpation (fingertip feel) they will sometimes find that a goiter is present (swelling) or that there are nodules within it. They can also feel the texture of the gland and whether it is unusually firm, when pressed upon. When a goiter is mild or nodules that are felt within the gland are small or several are found (single nodules are considered more suspicious than multiples), a doctor may not feel that further testing is merited. If however, a goiter is large enough to obstruct a patient's breathing or swallowing or if a thyroid nodule is large or very solid, imaging tests of the thyroid gland might then be ordered.

## Types of Thyroid Scans

Depending on the type of problem that is suspected to be affecting the thyroid gland, a doctor might order one or more of three types of tests. These would be "Thyroid Ultrasound", Radioactive Iodine Uptake Scan", CT Scan or an MRI (Magnetic Resonance Imaging).

## Ultrasound

With a Thyroid Ultrasound, a lab technician will use a small hand held device covered with a lubricating substance and they will run it across the front of the neck, in the area of the thyroid gland. A monitor will pick up sensitive sound waves that are sent to the thyroid gland and that return as an image on the screen (echo). This imaging will pick up a great amount of detail, including shapes and textures within the gland. The sonogram technology is the same as is used to monitor the fetuses of expectant mothers. While a continuous image will appear on the screen during this procedure, the technician can also take occasional still-images at the appropriate times, for review by medical doctors.

## Uptake Scan

A Radioactive Iodine Uptake Scan (RAIU) is an imaging test that utilizes radiology imaging, by giving the patient a carefully-measured dose of radioactive iodine. The substance is then absorbed by the thyroid gland, so that when imaging is taken, the tissue being observed will appear brighter and in more detail.

There are two basic purposes for thyroid uptake scans and often these are done in-combination, the one being to observe how much healthy thyroid tissue is present and capable of absorbing iodine and the other, to scan the imaging results for abnormal-looking thyroid tissue or nodules.

## CT Scan

A CT Scan (computed tomography or "cat scan) is a sophisticated type of x-ray imaging that takes images from a number of different angles simultaneously, so that the images can be compared for a more thorough evaluation than would simple x-rays that involve only one or two angle/views.

## MRI

An MRI is also an imaging method that will show greater detail but rather than only scanning the thyroid gland, it will also scan surrounding areas of the body and other glands related to thyroid function, such as the pituitary gland that is found in the brain (the origin of Thyroid Stimulating Hormone).

In the case of MRI, very powerful magnets are used to scan areas of the body to produce these detailed images and in some cases; a dose of an additional enhancer is given to patients, called "contrast" (gadolinium - a type of die).

## In Conclusion:

Thyroid testing is available to detect all forms and types of thyroid disorders and diseases, including imaging tests, tissue biopsy and blood analysis. If symptoms of thyroid hormone imbalance are being experienced or an abnormal size or texture is discovered within the gland (i.e. goiter and/or thyroid nodules), further evaluation by a qualified medical doctor is important and should not be delayed.

The vast majority of thyroid disease cases are successfully treated but timely diagnosis can be a key to better treatment outcomes.

**(END)**

## About the Author:

I am a husband, father, grandfather and lifetime contract salesman, with experience in health writing that began in 2004. I completed theological studies with Liberty University in 1996. I formerly served as editor and forum moderator of Thyroid Health for a major multi-topic content site and as a general health writer for another, where I achieved Editor's Choice Awards for my articles on health subjects.

In 2003 I was diagnosed with hypothyroidism; "Hashimoto's thyroiditis" being the cause. This autoimmune form of thyroid disease that causes destruction of the thyroid gland resulted in my also developing "Chronic Fatigue Syndrome", due to a compromised immune system with severe co-morbid "Adrenal Fatigue".

I also suffered severe anxiety symptoms, including panic attacks early into the onset of Hashimoto's thyroiditis (Hashitoxicosis). A common, benign heart murmur I was diagnosed with in my teens called "Mitral Valve Prolapse", also worsened in severity of symptoms, with the development of these other health disorders.

My eventual receiving of diagnoses was a difficult process with proper diagnostic testing not being ordered by the first doctors I sought treatment from. These types of issues were inspiration for me to become proactive in my own health care and to self-educate myself on these health disorders, which I have done extensively since 2003.

I now enjoy sharing this information with other patients experiencing my same health disorders.